# AYURVEDA

Happy for Life Using Traditional Principles of
Ayurveda

(Ayurvedic Healing for Beginners)

**Daniel Cummins**

Published by Knowledge Icons

**Daniel Cummins**

*Ayurveda: Happy for Life Using Traditional Principles of Ayurveda (Ayurvedic Healing for Beginners)*

ISBN 978-1-990084-80-5

**Legal & Disclaimer**

The information contained in this book is not designed to replace or take the place of any form of medicine or professional medical advice. The information in this book has been provided for educational and entertainment purposes only.

The information contained in this book has been compiled from sources deemed reliable, and it is accurate to the best of the Author's knowledge; however, the Author cannot guarantee its accuracy and validity and cannot be held liable for any errors or omissions. Changes are periodically made to this book. You must consult your doctor or get professional medical advice before using any of the

# TABLE OF CONTENTS

INTRODUCTION.................................................................1

CHAPTER 1: BEGINNERS' GUIDE TO AYURVEDA.................5

CHAPTER 2: AYURVEDIC ENERGY DRINKS WITH HERBS ... 14

CHAPTER 3: AYURVEDA REMEDIES FOR WEIGHT LOSS .... 22

CHAPTER 4: SIX TYPES OF TASTE IN FOOD CULTURE........ 28

CHAPTER 5: YOUR AYURVEDIC PHYSICAL AND MENTAL
CONSTITUTION.................................................................42

CHAPTER 6: AMLA GOOSEBERRY OF INDIAN DESCENT.... 50

CHAPTER 7: THE AYURVEDA DIET ....................................56

CHAPTER 8: WHAT IS THE FUNDAMENTAL REASONING OF
WELLBEING, SICKNESS AND TREATMENT IN AYURVEDA? 67

CHAPTER 9: AYURVEDA IN USE.........................................79

CHAPTER 10: THE AYURVEDIC WAY OF LIFE ...................91

CHAPTER 11: FIRM BREASTS.......................................... 105

CHAPTER 12: AYURVEDIC BODY TYPES .......................... 113

CHAPTER 13: WEIGHT LOSS........................................... 119

CHAPTER 14: AYYГNEdA ГEGIME FOГ WINTEГ dEPГESSION ................................................................. 130

CHAPTER 15: AYURVEDA AND INSOMNIA ..................... 135

CHAPTER 16: THE THREE DOŞAS ................................... 139

CHAPTER 17: A HEALTHY LIFE THROUGH THE AYURVEDA DIET ............................................................................ 149

# Introduction

Ayurveda is a system of Hindu medicine that has made a real tradition in the East and gradually it has also been adopted in many parts of the Western world as an additional means of approaching certain health problems, various aspects of lifestyle, and even a series of philosophical issues. Ayurveda practices are a form of alternative medicine which however were highly valued in the Hindu tradition. By no means was their importance considered to be secondary, given the strong belief in the healing properties of herbs and plants or of specific kinds of energy as well as in the power of white magic. Ayurveda dates from prehistoric times and has intersected with certain Vedic and non-Vedic systems and thus has assimilated aspects of other practices, too (e.g. Buddhism). By the Middle Ages, people who systematically practiced Ayurveda had already developed complex medicinal techniques and even surgical preparations.

The basis of Ayurveda is a holistic take on human health in which the physical and the mental dimensions strongly intertwine with individual personality in order to promote wellbeing. Thus practitioners of Ayurveda always consider all factors involved in a person's condition and try to treat illness by looking into the health of each side of one's existence. Ayurvedic doctors base their theories on the conviction that mind, matter, energy, and temperament highly influence one another and thus **any health problem should be approached holistically**, if healing is to be ensured. Although there are branches in Ayurveda that also deal with more complicated matters such as surgery, contemporary Ayurveda mainly centers on metabolism, healthy eating, meditation, yoga, energetic balance, and maintaining the optimal functioning of the digestive system (e.g. intake, excretion etc.).

Ayurveda also insists on **maintaining equilibrium** in all aspects of lifestyle such as sleep habits, relaxation, movement, activity/work, meditation/spiritual practices and so on. Once again, the holistic take on human health is quite remarkable, as psychological balance and physical wellbeing interweave in the basic principles of this medical practice. The main healing practices of Ayurveda are based on the power of cereals, plants, spices, and herbs. However there are also animal products that are encouraged in the diet that corresponds to Ayurvedic notions of health (e.g. milk or bones). According to the "rules" of Ayurveda, the whole metabolism and energetic balance of an individual should be carefully kept in check via diet for optimal health. In the following pages I will introduce you to the basics of Ayurveda. This guide to an old and valuable set of medical practices is meant to help beginners discover the essence of Ayurveda, the reasons why it should be included in one's life, and the best strategies and methods for assimilating Ayurvedic wisdom into one's lifestyle and mentality.

# Chapter 1: Beginners' Guide To Ayurveda

What is Ayurveda?

Put simply, Ayurveda is an ancient, traditional Hindu system of medicine, built on the belief that health depends on balance within certain bodily systems. It is considered by scholars to be the oldest healing science. "Ayu" is defined as life and "veda" means information. The basis of the science is that there must be harmony, a constant and healthy connection between the brain and the body.

It offers the opportunity for individuals to stay vibrant and vital. It allows you to fulfill your true human destiny. Through Ayurveda, you learn to create balance in your body and life. Freedom from illness depends on your own mindfulness, allowing your brain to bring your body into symmetry.

The History and Background of Ayurveda

The history of Ayurveda begins in the season of the Vedas, the ancient Holy Books of the Aryans. The scriptures, considered in the religion to be "not of man" and thus the most sacred of the texts, are thought to be the oldest of the Hindu literature, written 2,500-3,000 years ago. Hindu mythology holds that Lord Brahma, the maker of the world, passed on the teachings of Ayurveda to humankind. The four Vedas are called:

Rig Veda

Yajur Veda

Sama Veda

Atharva Veda

The standards of Ayurveda are based on these writings, particularly the Atharva Veda.

"Rishis" and "munis"—learned sages and holy people—dedicated their lives to discovering and discerning what made the world work. The words "rishi" and "muni" are interchangeable, however a rishi was often considered the more learned of the two. "Aryavarta", the name for Northern India in Sanskrit literature, encompassed the Himalayas, and was considered to be home to the rishis and munis. In present-day, the area includes the nations of Nepal, India, Pakistan, Bhutan, and Bangladesh.

In mythological terms, the Vedas tell the stories of Indra, the leader of the Devas and Deva of rain and thunderstorms; of the Ashwini, the first lunar mansion of Hindu astrology; and Prajapati, the "lord of people" reigning over procreation and protection of life—a "King of Kings"—among others. They tell the tale of Ayurveda's otherworldly beginnings, detailing the exchange of knowledge between the divine creatures and the sages.

Principles of Ayurveda

Essential Principles of Ayurveda contain:

Three Fundamental all-inclusive energies

Satva

Rajas

Tamas

The PancaMahabhutas and its five essential components

Akasha: space.

Vayu: air.

Teja or Agni: fire.

Jala: water.

Prithviwhich: earth.

The TriDosas—Three Body Humours

Vata

Pitta

Kapha

The Sapta Dhatus—Seven Types of body tissues

Rasa Dhatu (liquid)

Rakta Dhatu (blood)

Mamsa Dhatu

Meda Dhatu  (fat)

Asthi Dhatu

Majja Dhatu

Sukra Dhatu

The TrayodosaAgni—Three Types of digestive flames

Jatharagni (gastric flame)

Sapta Dhatvagni

Panca Bhutagni

The TriMalas—Three Types of Body Wastes

Purisa: feces.

Mutra: urine.

Sveda: sweat.

Components of Ayurveda—"Ashtanga Ayurveda"

The eight components of Ayurveda are known collectively as "Ashtanga Ayurveda". They are:

General Medicine

Pediatrics

Psychology

Ophthalmology

Surgery

Toxicology

Rejuvenation Therapy

Reproductive Medicine

General Medicine

This first branch of Ayurveda is known as the "Kaaya Chikitsa" or literally "Body Treatment". This branch primarily manages the analysis and treatment of general sicknesses. It is fundamentally the treatment of the entire body, from something as minor as skin infections to something as deadly as tuberculosis.

Pediatrics

This branch encompasses everything identified with children, including the procedure of child bearing. From pre-natal to perinatal, conception to embryo development, nutrition for pregnant women, this branch covers it all. After birth, it deals all aspects of new-born and youth healthcare.

Psychology

This branch manages the psyche and its illnesses. As per Ayurveda, numerous mantras and yogis can condition one to thereby cure mental illness. The belief is that it is the wrong use of the mind that causes mental instability.

Ophthalmology

This branch deals with the diagnoses and treatment of diseases of the eye.

Surgery

Anything from tumors to complicated deliveries can be taken care of utilizing the Ayurvedic strategies of this branch.

Toxicology

This branch deals with the cleansing of one's body of the various contaminants and toxins we are exposed to every day.

Rejuvenation Therapy

This branch deals with the maintenance of one's good health, mind and body, so that there is continuing balance and harmony.

Reproductive Medicine

This branch manages fertility concerns, not just with humans but also plants and animals.

How Ayurveda is different from Modern-day Medicine

The contrast between Ayurvedic medicine and Modern medicine is most basic. Modern medicine treats the symptoms or after-effects of the illness. Ayurveda treats the whole body, from prevention to maintenance.

Say you feel sick with what you think is the flu. The first thing you might do is go to the doctor where you have your temperature taken, maybe some tests are ordered and then you are prescribed a medication that carries with it some kind of side-effect warnings. The infection is treated but the reason for it is not addressed in full.

Ayurveda desires to dispense with the main reason for—the root cause of—the ailment so that the body is returned to a strong, healthy state and no side effects linger. It strives to provide a cure, not a temporary fix. It works to rid the illness, restore the body and mind to health and then employ preventative measures to ensure no further problems arise. The theory is you have only one body for your entire life, so it's best to treat it well with the goal that it will serve you well.

Ayurvedic medicine utilizes plants and herbs to accomplish its ends. Unlike modern medicine, based on man-made chemical compounds, there are no lingering side-effects. Modern medicine often creates more problems, even after the initial illness has been treated.

## Chapter 2: Ayurvedic Energy Drinks With Herbs

While Ayurveda deals with the digestion of the whole body and makes a connection and balance between our mind, body and spirit, it also mentions some instructions to be followed. It is very necessary to initiate our day with a proper well focused mind and in good spirit, with a positive frame of mind. Ayurveda also suggests making an early start to your morning. That is to wake up early in the morning when only a few rays of sun scatter the clouds. This way Ayurveda suggests is beneficial to the body. In this chapter we have mentioned a few Ayurveda energy drinks with some fresh herbs incorporated to keep the body healthy. Not only will we mention the drinks name but you can also find their recipes so as to know how to exactly make them. Some of them are:

1. Cinnamon, almond and date shake:

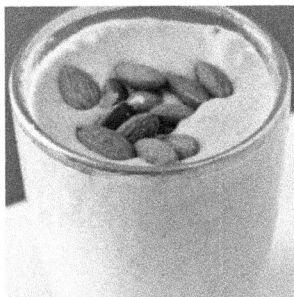

One of the best things about this drink is that it takes a very little amount of time to prepare it, hardly 6 to 7 minutes. And also this drink can be prepared for breakfast when the stomach is empty. This way the first thing consumed by the body will be a healthy drink which will ease up the digestion process. This shake has a combination of two flavors, the sweet and the spice. While the dates add sweetness to the shake making your mind and body relax, your mood better, the cinnamon adds up some spice and comforting the body.

This drink removes any kind of exhaustion daunting your body and dates are known for calming the nerves of a person. Apart from this, dates and almond are a good combination to give strength to the liver and to control the emotions and give them comfort. Not only this both date and almond are ojas building tonics. Ojas is an ayurvedic term used when a person has good healthy body. So indirectly this drink boosts calmness, perseverance, and peace to the mind. Its ingredients include milk, almond, dates, cinnamon and ginger.

2. Fennel, coriander and cumin tea

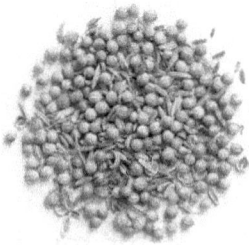

This drink includes the fresh herb called the coriander. It is basically a type of tea.

So it's best for those who like tea. This drink is easy and simple to make and is known for its usefulness in promoting weight loss and helping in detoxification. According to the ayurvedic concept this drink helps the runny nose and the flu, the cough trying to finish the congestion swelling up in the mucus. This drink speeds up the metabolism process and aids in the purificating of the blood.

It eases ones nerves, and prevents any kind of inflammation or swelling. In order to get the best results one must drink this at least 3 to 4 times a day. It is extra ordinary simple to make. The only thing required is a hot cup of water and add in the three ingredients. Stir it, and there you go. As this drink is mostly dilute, containing majority of water into it it is advisable not to drink it before sleeping as it will cause the drinker the trouble of having to urinate again and again.

3. Ashwagandha

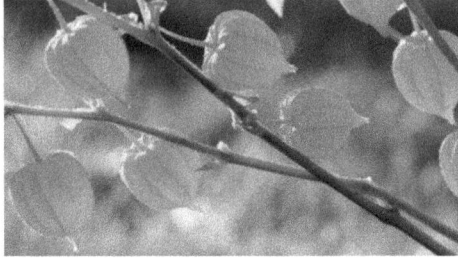

This is a natural ayurvedic herb which is used in ayurvedic medicines known for solving problems related to extreme weakness, lethargic conditions and to relieve one from exhaustion. This herb makes a person's immune strong enough not to let stress overcome them and also improves the level of energy. The term ashwaganda in the sanskrit means "smell of the horse" which clearly indicates the valour, determination and strength of the horse.

This herb originates from a short shrub, with leaves of oval shape and yellow flowers. This herb grows in mild climates for example mostly in India, Middle East and now even in the United States. Apart from relieving the stress and building the immunity of the body strong this herb has some other benefits also such as it enhances the sex drive of both the men and the women. It also lowers the cholesterol level, reduces the risk of malaria, keeps a balanced blood sugar level, prevents depression, and develops the IQ level of the brain also.

4. Ojas drink

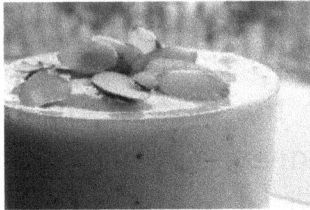

Ojas is related to the seven tissues in our body. It is related with the immunity, and energy of the body. It is said that the one having ojas in their system finds it much easier to fight against diseases. It also acts as an anti ageing system. This drink also contains ginger, and its countless benefits we have already explained in the remaining chapters. This drink can be prepared quite quickly and the ingredients needed are as follows. Almonds, water, dates, raised petals, ghee, few saffron strands, cardamom, dry powdered ginger, and honey.

In this drink, the almonds need to be blanched, and the dates also need to be soaked in water to make them tender over the night. Put these in a blender and blend them until they form a thick consistency. Then add in the blender the rose petals, the ghee, honey, saffron, cardamom and ginger. Blend all of these until they form into what should look like a drink. This drink should be consumed twice or thrice in a week. This drink will work wonders. One can only think this by looking at such amazing ingredients it has. All these ingredients are readily and easily available in every supermarket and even in your home. People who have increased number of toxins should avoid this drink.

## Chapter 3: Ayurveda Remedies For Weight Loss

If you want to reduce weight, you can use Ayurvedic medicine because it is close to modern medications. Both modern and Ayurveda are agreed that the obesity is caused just because of an imbalance between calorie expenditure and intake. You have to follow a healthy eating and exercise routine to fight with obesity. With Ayurveda, you can cure obesity and remove stubborn fat of your body without any painful surgery. The ayurvedic cure for obesity has three cleft approaches.

First: You have to use herbs to reduce weight to mobilize stubborn fat of your body.

Second: Carefully constructs one diet plan to reduce your weight.

Third: Make one exercise schedule, stick to this schedule and manage a healthy weight.

If anyone tells you that their medicine will help you to reduce weight without dieting and exercise, they are just lying to you.

Natural Ingredients

There are numerous ayurvedic medicines to treat your obesity and melt excessive fat of your body without any side effect. You can use natural ingredients without any fear or potential side effects. These are better than arterial weight loss pills because these are free from any side effects. Some common Ayurvedic medications for obesity are as under.

Ginger

It is a common ingredient easily found in your kitchen, and you can use it to reduce weight. This natural item is an important part of ayurvedic medications for obesity. It is good to treat your metabolism, stimulate oxidation of all fatty acids in your body and reduce the cholesterol levels in your blood.

Kalonji

Kalonji aka Nigella sativa works well to reduce a good amount of weight. This seed helps you to maintain ideal body mass. This black seed is good to reduce your aging process and prevent osteoporosis. It is scientifically approved that Kalonji can boost your metabolism, clear your airways and increase the strength of your immune system.

Guggul

This Ayurveda medication works really well to improve cholesterol in your body and help you to reduce weight. Guggul is a common flowering tree, and it can protect you from numerous diseases. It is an important part of Ayurveda medications to lower cholesterol, detoxify the body, purify your blood, maintain a safe cholesterol levels, promote healthy weight and support your immune system.

Licorice

This ingredient is good for your liver and increases the quality of your blood. You can reduce weight without bearing any physical or mental stress. It is good to soothe your stomach and repair the lining of your belly. It is good to reduce stress, treat the problems of your respiratory system and protect your teeth and skin.

Home Remedies to Reduce Weight

You can follow different efficient remedies to shed extra pounds. Some of these remedies are as under.

Start your day with a glass of lukewarm water and squeeze one lemon into this glass. Drink it on an empty stomach.

Fast on lime juice and honey to detoxify your body and improve your metabolism.

Soak one teaspoon of cumin seeds and carom seeds in one glass of water and leave it for one night. Boil this concoction in the morning until the water reduced to half and drink it early morning. Drink this water on a regular basis and prevent retention of water in your body.

Ayurvedic Herbs

There are some incredible herbs to fight against stubborn weight and cholesterol in your body. These will help you to shed a good amount of body fat.

Aloe Vera

It has numerous health benefits, but weight loss is its exclusive property. You can drink a glass of Aloe Vera juice to reduce extra fat from your body. You can make an herbal mix with aloe vera, haritiki, giloy and cumin seeds. You can mix some honey in this mixture and use it in the early morning with your empty stomach.

Curry Powder and Curry Leaves

Curry powder and curry leaves both are good to reduce weight. You can Boil curry leaves in water and drink this brew in the morning. You can chew fresh leaves to shed extra body fat. These leaves have a good impact on your estrogen.

Curry powder is good to consume on a regular basis in salads and soups. The curry powder is made of fenugreek seeds, cinnamon, cloves, coriander seeds, cumin seeds, and turmeric powder. You can combine all spices in equal quantity and use this powerful mix to melt your body fat.

Mint

It is incredibly powerful to stimulate your gallbladder to release extra bite. You can make chutney with mint, curry leaves, and coriander. Enhance the taste of this chutney with some lemon juice and salt. You can include this condiment (chutney) in your diet and see its visible impacts on your health.

You can use these items during ayurvedic treatment, but make sure to follow a healthy diet. A healthy diet, good exercise routine, and herbal remedies prove good to shed your extra body fat.

# Chapter 4: Six Types Of Taste In Food Culture

These basic tastes can be observed in our everyday diet due to every taste has different elemental composition, it is very essential to pay much closer attention to some details of them.

| Taste | Composition | Examples |
|---|---|---|
| Sweet(Madur) | Earth and Water | Mango, Banana |
| Sour(Amla) | Earth and Fire | Lemon, Orange |
| Salty(Lavan) | Water and Fire | Sea Salt |
| Pungent(Thik) | Air and Fire | Ginger, Black Pepper |
| Bitter(Katu) | Air and Space | **Neem** |

| Astringent(Kased ) | Air and Earth | Guava, Lentils |
|---|---|---|

Deep body place with action of Vata, Pitta, Kapha in body: -

| Energy/Dosha | Deep Body Place | Balanced action | Imbalanced action |
|---|---|---|---|
| Vata | Lungs, Nervous System | Respiration, Movements of body parts, Nerve energy conduction | Paralysis, Joint Pain, nerve disorder, stress |
| Pitta | Stomach, Pancreas, Heart | Digestion, heat regulation, | Acidity, Skin Disease, Heart |

|  |  | complexion, aura | problem, uric acid. |
|---|---|---|---|
| **Kapha** | Saliva, Intestinal Juices, Lubrication of Joint Fluids | Immunity, Lubrication, Strength and organ protection | Asthma, Laziness, Fatigue. |

Healing through Tastes: -

| Taste | Composition and effective Dosha | Useful In these situation | Herbs Used |
|---|---|---|---|
| **Sweet** | Water and Earth(Kapha) | Weakness, lack of energy, stamina | **Ashwagandha** |
| **Sour** | Earth and | Loss of | Lemon, |

| | Fire (Kapha, pitta) | appetite | Orange |
|---|---|---|---|
| **Salty** | Fire and Water (Pitta, Kapha) | Indigestion, cramps | Sea Salt |
| **Pungent** | Air and Fire (Vata, Pitta) | Diabetes, obesity, lethargy | Pepper, Ginger |
| **Bitter** | Air and Space(Vata) | Skin problem, obesity | Neem, Bitter gourd |
| **Astringent** | Air and Earth (Vata, Kapha) | Heavy Bleeding | **Ashoka** |

Another information related to meal for calculative diet: -

Divide your stomach in four parts virtually then take solid food for 50%, 25% salads &

fruits and keep 25% vacant for regulation of all essential digestive air to flow easily which reduce chances of acidity and heaviness.

If we take all our meals in this proportion according to our body type with respect to time of dosha in daytime then it's very hard to get ill without any major reasons.

Herbs: -

Herbs should always intake according to nature of body because every person is combination of different prakriti and doshas.

Ayurveda looks at holistic healing of a person not just of the body but also of mind and emotional energy as well it is basically related with tridosha and their balance that's what said leads to the optimum health of a person if a particular dosha specially the pre-dominant one becomes aggravated then it leads to certain health issues.

We already give you little bit information about vata types so let's talk about how to calm these dosha with the element of space and air vata dosha is responsible for all activities of body and mind when dosha becomes aggravated it may lead to anxiety, insomnia and digestive issue.

So, let's talk about some herbs which are good for pre-dominant vata dosha and then to keep it in balance.

Ashwagandha

This is known as Indian ginseng has a taste of sweet, bitter and astringent contains heating effect for body, it is very good rejuvenating herb for coping stress and previously damaged cell within the system.

Other benefits of it is imparting vigor, strengthen the immune system, claim nervous system and helps the mind in focusing better with enhancement of physical power within the system.

Triphala

This has a taste of sweet, sour, bitter pungent as well as astringent has a heating and cooling effect on the body and the mind.

Triphala is the combination of bibhitiki, amalki and haritaki which is dried to make powder in specific proportion of these herbs.

Helps in cleansing and detoxifies the body, nourishment of bones which can be very dry in people with an aggravated vata dosha to strengthens the immunity system.

Ginger

Herb has pungent taste with heating effect on the body, anti-inflammatory phytonutrients called gingerols.

Improves digestion, helps getting rid of nausea, cold & flu which vata people is very much prone to and also Helps to stabilize metabolism of system.

If you have aggravated vata then these herbs including in your diet will help you to get rid of vata dosha imbalance.

Pitta

Imbalance of this dosha can leads to many problems related to digestion as well as metabolism because after all pitta dosha is responsible for various function of digestion as well as metabolism.

So, some herbs related to balance pitta are given below, let's have a look

Bacopa (Brahmi)

This has taste of sweet and bitter with cooling effect on the body, helps body to cope with stress and anxiety, alleviates depression and helps in having sound sleep.

Helps to Cools down mind to making it calmer to reduce effect of aggravated pitta dosha, curing ulcer and other GI tract issue which can leads to various infection also other ill health issues.

Triphala

As discussed earlier due to mixture of three fruits dried and mixed together this herb is beneficial for every body type because this contains heating and cooling both effects for system if used properly this can-do miracle on your digestive health situation.

So just like you know herb has taste of sweet, sour, bitter pungent as well as astringent has a heating and cooling effect on the body and the mind.

Triphala is very much beneficial for regulating digestive fire in body and helps to keep it in vibrant condition which is essential for healthy body because if stomach gets upset it makes body prone to every kind of illness.

Helps in cleansing and detoxifies the body, nourishment of digestive fire which can be very hot in people with an aggravated pitta dosha to strengthens the immunity system.

Shatavar

herb should be used in calculated quantity by people who are prone to pitta dosha because this herb is also used for vata people to gain strength and immunity for muscle gaining efficiently and herb also has sweet and bitter taste with hot and cooling effect on the body, elevate heartburn and gastric issues which pitta people are very much prone to

Helps in cases of irritable bowel syndrome and UTI with avoiding irritability by claiming the mind.

Pitta dosha can be controlled by using these herbs in your daily food habits and can be used as powerful medicine to cure various types of disease.

You will see difference in your physical and mental health if you religiously make them part of your diet and life.

**Kapha**

Majority of people gets effected by these dosha irrespective of their body type so keeping this dosha in proper balance is very important for all types of bodies.

Turmeric (Haldi)

This has a pungent bitter and astringent taste and one of the most potent herb in curing various types of aliments within the system contains heating effect for body which is important to balance the kapha dosha.

Helps in detoxifying body, protects liver with soothing effect on the digestive system, powerful anti-inflammatory and anti-oxidant properties.

Triphala

Herb with taste of sweet, sour, bitter pungent as well as astringent has a heating and cooling effect on the body and the mind.

Helps in cleansing and detoxifies the body, controlled nourishment of bones and lubrication of body tissues which can be very beneficial for people with an aggravated kapha dosha to strengthens the immunity system.

Ginger

This has pungent taste with heating effect on body and improve digestive capacity of human system, Reducing and curing cold & flu to stabilize metabolism.

This herb is also used as very potent medicine for various types of other disease related to enhancement of ojha to cure bones & skin problems of vata and kapha people

Yoga: -

It is very wide science used to aligned physical, mental, emotional and energy system of our body properly focused in one direction so we can manifest whatever we want in our life easily.

Before talking about it we can look at some situations that we face and observe everyday related to our physical, mental, emotional habits so let's look at some questions

Why we look like our parent?

Why we react in different situations in same way?

Why we hang around so much between past memory and future imagination?

So, if we just look at these few questions which moves us toward finding out some answer related to our reoccurring physical, mental and emotional habits and without going into too much details of it, I will make it as simple as I can.

There is various system of yoga to take control of different habits of your sub conscious mind programming and help you in re programming of your sub consciously written programmed to mind with body.

some of these systems to help you in mind and body reprogramming are

Gyan Yoga

Mantra yoga

Laya yoga

Hatha yoga

Karma yoga

Bhakti yoga

Raj yoga or Ashtanga yoga

## Chapter 5: Your Ayurvedic Physical And Mental Constitution

In Ayurveda, one's physical and mental constitution is already pre- determined at birth and the qualities or dominances of the combination of one's tri dosha (vita, Pitta, Kapha) are unique to every individual.

A person's Kapha sums up the water in his body and determines his flesh quality and secretions.

His Pitta, on the other hand gives warmth to his body and transforms substances like plasma.

Lastly, his Vata determines energies and activities needed for a healthy balance of his doshas.

However, it is inevitable that one humor is dominant than the others. This dominance marks one's uniqueness in terms of disposition and physical appearance.

From an Ayurvedic perspective, optimum health may be achieved by first knowing by heart one's natural constitution in order to know the first step in any treatment. One's predominant humor greatly reflects the qualities and make-up of an individual. The belief is that, most diseases arise from the predominant biological humor of an individual. In general, having knowledge of this and knowing how and what to balance is the main key in optimizing one's health. This process gives Ayurveda the ability to prevent disease, maintain health and maximize lifespan.

The Vata Constitution

Individuals of Vata constitution are generally considered to be physically underdeveloped. They are usually light with flexible, small-framed bodies and with chests that are flat making their tendons and veins visible. Individuals under this constitution tend to have less stamina and strength than the other types.

Vatas generally have dry and rough skin and cold hands and feet. This is so because of their poor circulation. They also have the tendency to experience indigestion and crave for sweet, sour and salty taste and hot drinks. They also perspire much less than the other types. Their production of sweat and urine is scanty, even their feces is dry and hard.

Vatas always seem to be in a rush. They dislike the idea of sitting for long hours and prefer constant activity. Psychologically, Vatas are gifted with quick mindedness, creativity and excellent imagination. They also have the tendency to talk a lot and generally have a quite loving and sweet personality. Fear is the most prominent manifestation of imbalance in Vatas. This is the reason why they are also susceptible to anxiety attacks, nervousness and loneliness.

To help maintain balance in Vata constitution, the following are advised:

Dress warmly

Avoid cold food

Avoid raw food

Keep a routine/daily habit

Try to stay calm/ be aware of impulsiveness

Try to stay away from extreme cold temperatures

The Pitta Constitution

Pitta individuals also have the tendency to have flat chests but unlike Vatas, their veins and tendons have a medium prominence. They usually have a slender built and their body frame seems delicate to look at but their bones are not as prominent like the Vatas. Their bones are not as underdeveloped as the Vatas. They tend to have a lot of moles and freckles which are brownish or reddish in color. The Pitta complexion is usually fair, reddish or coppery while their skin is soft and warm to touch. Physiologically, pitas have a strong metabolism. As a result, they have a good appetite and good digestion and they tend to eat and drink a lot. Pittas also have the tendency to perspire a lot, thus making their body temperature slightly higher, making their hands and feet warm.

Physiologically, pitas tend to have diseases related to the fire element or heat. Inflammation, colitis, heart burn, jaundice, and sore throats and 'itis-related' diseases are examples of manifestations of imbalance in a Pitta constitution. Psychologically, Pitta individuals are gifted with good concentration and comprehension. They are generally considered intellects with good logical thinking and sharp memories. Pittas are good speakers, great leaders and have a great capacity for organizing. As a matter of fact, they also have a lot of charisma that attracts people which turns them to professions like politicians, lawyers, doctors and other noble professions, During an imbalance, Pittas have the tendency to criticize, judge and to be perfectionists.

This is why Pitta individuals tend to have moderate lifespans because they burn their life energy through mental activity.

To help maintain the balance in the Pitta constitution, the following are recommended:

Preferring cooling /bland or non-spicy food

Drinking cool drinks but not overly iced

Avoiding too much salty and oily food

Exercising during the cooler part of the day

The Kapha Constitution

The Kapha individual, unlike the other two previously discussed constitutions, is blessed with a developed, strong and healthy body. Their chests are prominent, well-developed and have strong muscles. Their body frame is large due to the dominance of earth and water elements in their constitution so they tend to be mostly healthy and strong. Kaphas also have strong, white teeth and hair that is soft, lustrous and thick. Although their metabolism is not as fast as the Pittas, Kaphas can go on with their day while skipping their meals. But because of their slow metabolic rate, Kaphas tend to have a longer lifespan. They also prefer sweets and salty tastes.

Psychologically, Kaphas tend to feel heavy and foggy in the mornings for they are midday people. Kaphas tend to move a bit slow and are often lethargic. They move slow-paced and their speech pattern is monotonous. When there is imbalance, obesity, diabetes, water retention are the manifestations. But when there is balance, Kaphas are caring, compassionate, patient and tolerant.

To maintain balance in the Kapha constitution, the following are recommended:

Prefer dry and light food, avoid heavy food

Keep active and get plenty of exercise

Avoid dairy

Keep routine

## Chapter 6: Amla Gooseberry Of Indian Descent.

Amla is known for many health benefits, being one of the essential foods in Ayurvedic medicine. Amla berry is the king of antioxidants in wholefood, containing more antioxidants than every other wholefood. Amla has the highest vitamin C content in plant life at 720 mg per 100 g.

Although it tastes very bitter and sour, Amla is commonly used as fresh fruit and in herbal medicine for culinary purposes in India. As modern science has been looking into this superfood's fantastic health benefits, Amla is gaining prominence and renown in the Western World.

Amla is a renowned superfood that guards the liver, acidity balances, improves fertility, and enhances overall health. The fruit can also combat ulcers, as it can inhibit gastric acid development while encouraging mucus secretion.

Amla has multiple applications for therapy. This has antioxidants, antibacterial properties, anti-inflammatory properties, and anti-cancer properties. Science has shown that by activating the active killer cells, eating Amla enhances immunity. Amla is effective in reducing stress and toning the nervous system; its anti-aging property helps preserve function in the kidneys. As a cardiovascular tonic, Amla reduces cholesterol by stimulating decomposition and inhibiting inadequate cholesterol production, and daily Amla intake also reduces arterial plaque making it a robust cardiovascular ally.

Amla 's beneficial strength lies in both the high levels of polyphenolic compounds it produces and ascorbic acid. Amla is probably the most abundant source of ascorbic acid (Vitamin C) that exists in its most active bioform. Efficient antioxidants are polyphenols such as emblicanine and amla-containing ascorbic acid. Oxidative stress is a chronic phenomenon in our bodies. This cycle is increased both with age and due to external factors such as noise, physical exertion, etc. This oxidative stress cycle is responsible for the creation of free radicals. Such free radicals are the antioxidants within the amla mop.

The presence of emblicanins in Amla (hence the scientific name Emblica Officinalis) is what makes Amla a special and perhaps the most potent antioxidant. Emblicanin has the properties of pro oxidation. When any antioxidant such as vitamin E or vitamin A, beta carotene, etc. mops up the free radicals, these healthy antioxidant molecules are turned into free radicals themselves, which can, in fact, cause longer-term oxidative damage. In the case of Amla, the antioxidant Emblicanin A checks and destroys the free radicals aggressively. If a free radical is neutralized, it is then converted into Emblicanin B, which is again an antioxidant. Amla is thus capable of moping up the full volume of free radicals.

Amla is considered to be much more durable than antioxidants such as green tea, resveratrol, vitamin C, the extract of grape seeds and extract of pine. A high intake of Amla provides defense against erythrocyte disintegration (red blood cells). This could have immense significance as red blood cell disintegration can lead to myriad diseases, from heart failure to renal failure.

Amla's benefits.

Amla may not be pleasant in taste but is still a little bag full of antioxidants that help a lot for your body. This has the highest vitamin C content of all fruits and vegetables. It is also an outstanding detoxifying agent and supports boost immunity. Early morning is the best time to consume amla, particularly during the winters whenever the temperature drops. It eliminates unnecessary toxins from the body and is a potential source of nutrients vitamin C and calcium, in addition to cleaning the colon. Amla is also considered to be protective against dandruff, and other issues with skincare.

Vitamin C: Amla has eight times as much vitamin C as peach, twice as much antioxidant as acai berry and about 17 times more than pomegranate. Similar to store-bought supplements, vitamin C in amla is absorbed more quickly by the body. What you can do is mix 2 teaspoons of amla powder with two teaspoons of honey and have it for instant relief three to four times a day when you have a cold or cough, or drink it once daily for regular safety.

Builds immunity: Antioxidants and vitamin C in amla also help improve immunity and avoid viral and bacterial illnesses, including cold and cough. While amla juice can be a tad unpalatable, it is incredibly beneficial. It can also be eaten as a treat, made with a mixture of amla, jaggery, and rock salt. Two-three dumplings can be fed directly after meals.

Aids digestion: Amla helps to pass the bowels healthily by keeping the gastrointestinal tract clean. This effectively avoids rising digestive problems like constipation. We can also regulate acidity and indigestion with amla. Some relief can be provided by a half teaspoon of amla powder with a glass of warm water.

Perfect for hair and skin: Amla works as a hair tonic. This combats premature graying, prevents dandruff, strengthens hair follicles and improves the circulation of blood to the scalp, thereby increasing hair growth. Amla is the most energetic fruit, which is anti-aging. Each morning drinking amla juice with honey will give you flawless, clean, and glowing skin.

Diabetes: Amla helps the body respond to insulin as a great source of chromium, which helps to regulate insulin sensitivity. It helps to regulate blood sugar levels and can be consumed as part of your diet. However, daily diabetes medicine is no substitute for this.

## Chapter 7: The Ayurveda Diet

When it comes to the Ayurveda diet, you don't have to think that you'll be constantly eating only vegetables, rice and legumes. The diet's fundamental principles are applicable to any cuisine, be it Asian, Mediterranean, European, or any other cuisine.

The saying 'You are what you eat' holds true on a physical and psychological level. When your diet mostly consists of French fries and hamburgers, you may probably feel like French fries and hamburgers—and not in a good way. In the Ayurveda diet, it is essential that your foods are fresh, organic, local and seasonal. However, fresh doesn't always mean 'raw'. What you should consume are whole, freshly-cooked meals.

Cook more often with fresh produce. Use some of the basic Ayurveda spices like coriander, cumin, ginger and turmeric. You can add the spices to any dish that you cook. Aside from being excellent digestion and flavor enhancers, Ayurveda spices can also offer medicinal benefits.

Benefits of the Ayurveda Diet

Ailment Cure. The Ayurveda principles state that to cure all health-related problems, it is crucial to change the patient's diet. The combination of Ayurveda dietary rules and the right supplements is believed to cure any health issue.

Healthy Weight. The Ayurveda diet can help you achieve a healthy and normal weight—without getting too thin. Many contemporary weight loss plans and fads damage the body by depleting or burning nutrients—not only excess fat. The Ayurveda diet promotes eating foods according to a person's dosha. Additionally, individuals suffering from anorexia can also use the Ayurveda diet to be healthier.

Increased Life Span. When you follow the Ayurveda diet, you achieve balance among the doshas. You can expect your mind and body to function at their best. The diet also helps to create new cells and enhances your existing cells'survival period. When your cells function efficiently, you live a healthier and longer life.

Increased Energy. In Ayurveda, the digestive system is believed to be the body's main energy source. The first effect is on your digestive system as you eat. After achieving balance, your body's energy blocks are released, thereby ensuring a better energy flow.

Personalized for your Dietary Needs. The Ayurveda is based on the six tastes, including astringent, bitter, sour, salty, sweet and pungent. It's also based on the six food qualities like heavy/light, hot/cold, and oily/dry. Some of the tastes and qualities increase any of the three doshas (vata, pitta, and kapha), while others work in decreasing them.

Each person's diet varies accordingly, and you are free to choose any food according to the qualities and tastes. It is easier for you to manage it then, and you have a number of foods to choose from.

Reduces Ama. In Ayurveda, the term 'ama' means toxicity, which works against 'agni.' When your 'agni' (digestive fire) is low, your body is not capable of properly digesting food. This leads to ama (toxin) production in your body.

Six Tastes in the Ayurveda Diet

Ayurveda distinguishes six tastes and you should have all of them in your everyday diet. They are:

Sweet—milk, pasta, rice, honey, sugar, etc.

Sour—vinegar, yogurt, hard cheese, lemons, etc.

Salty—salt or any food that contains salt

Pungent—ginger, cayenne, chili peppers, any hot spice

Bitter—lettuce, turmeric, leafy greens, etc.

Astringent–lentils, beans, pomegranate, etc.

The six tastes are in the order that your body digests them. Any sweets or carb dish you eat gets digested first, thus, it is advisable to eat your dessert at the beginning of your meal. On the other hand, you need to eat salad as you end your meal.

Integrating all the six tastes in the Ayurveda diet contributes to a feeling of fullness at the end of each meal. As such, cravings are usually caused by not having the six tastes in your meals. A lot of people often omit the astringent and bitter tastes, even when both tastes are important. When you are eating something astringent or bitter at the end of your meal, you reduce your craving to eat desserts.

In the Ayurveda diet, integrating the six tastes improves your health immensely. You also get to lose some unwanted weight effortlessly

Agni

In the Ayurveda diet, agni (digestive fire) is considered the most important concept by Ayurveda practitioners and physicians. You can digest whatever you consume when your agni is strong and healthy. When your digestive fire is weak, you are unable to digest your food and your body easily produces toxins.

For agni balance, try to eat lightly and follow some healthy eating habits. You may include ginger tea in your diet. Peel and grate¼inch of ginger. Pour hot water over it and allow it to sit for 5 minutes. Sip the tea daily.

Eating Out

The practice of eating outside the home is prevalent throughout the world, especially if you don't want to cook your own meals or if you don't have the time to prepare your meals after work. However, you can still follow the Ayurveda diet as long as you know some basic tips when it comes to dining out.

The first and important pointer on eating out is to ask for warm or room temperature water, instead of cold water with lots of ice. Nothing kills the agni (digestive fire) faster than drinking cold water on an empty stomach.

Keep in mind the quality and tastes of food when you dine out. If you are armed with the knowledge on what qualities and tastes balance your Ayurveda body type, you can make the right food choices.

If your dosha is predominantly pitta, you will do fine if you eat at salad bars and eat mostly raw food. You may also eat vegetarian dishes. Avoid eating tomato, garlicky and deep fried dishes. Know that anything spicy/hot aggravates pitta.

If your dosha is predominantly vata, it is best to favor warm soup over a cold salad. When dining out, avoid cold, raw foods and concentrate more on warm, well-cooked dishes.

If your dosha is predominantly kapha, you should do well to eat light food items like light vegetarian dishes and lightly cooked/steamed vegetables. Avoid dishes that are oily/heavy and those that are fried and have lots of sour cream or cheese.

Healthy Eating Habits

If you take note of some healthy habits and favor healthy foods for your dominant dosha, you can augment your digestion and experience immense health benefits.

Eating should be a cherished ritual. Before eating, say grace or take three to five slow breaths. Such process can prepare you to receive food.

Eat food that is lovingly prepared. The cook's energy is in the food, therefore, you need to avoid eating dishes made by a resentful cook. In Ayurveda, not only do you eat food, you also take in the cook's emotions.

Eat in a calm place. Don't eat with the radio or television turned on. Don't even read. Also, engage in limited conversation and don't talk about emotionally intense subject matters.

Chew your food well. As you eat, be mindful of the food in your mouth. Properly chewing your food improves absorption and digestion.

Eat with a moderate pace until you are three-quarters full. One of society's major disease causes is overeating. As you eat a lot of food, your digestion suffers. After you have finished eating, you should no longer feel hungry and heavy.

Don't drink a lot of liquids with your meals. Half a cup of room temp water is acceptable. You don't have to drink liquids with moist meals. However, in eating dry meals, you may need to drink more. Take all your drinks, including water, warm or at room temperature as cold drinks decrease digestion by destroying the digestive fire.

Allow 15 to 20 minutes to digest your food. After eating your meal, rest a bit and allow your food to digest before doing other things. By this, read a book or have a conversation with your eating companion. You can also take a walk. Take at least three to five breaths as a culmination of your meal.

Let your meals digest for at least three hours. This means, you can take 3 to 5 meals a day.

Make lunch as your heaviest meal. The smallest should be your dinner. Your body digests food best at around lunchtime when the sun is high. The rhythm of the body mirrors the universe's rhythm. Also, you need to eat breakfast. Eat a larger breakfast if you are famished. If not, drink ginger tea as an appetite stimulate, so you can have even a small breakfast.

While losing excess fat and normalizing body weight is a great side effect of following the Ayurveda diet, it is even more important to know that Ayurveda's goal is to bring you back to your true constitution. It is also important to restore balance in your mind and body. Ayurveda takes you back to your real nature where you experience happiness, balance and optimal health.

## Chapter 8: What Is The Fundamental Reasoning Of Wellbeing, Sickness And Treatment In Ayurveda?

According to Ayurveda, "Wellbeing" is a condition of harmony of ordinary elements of Dooshas, Dhatus, malas and Agni with pleased body, psyche and soul. It implies that when Dosh-Dhatu-Malas and Agni are continually in a condition of practical balance, then the wellbeing is kept up. Generally twisting of the balance comes about into infections. Inconsistent way of life is accepted to be one of the essential causes behind the disappointment of system of looking after balance.

Treatment either with or without medications and utilization of particular tenets of eating regimen, movement and mental status as depicted, illness insightful, brings back the condition of harmony i.e. wellbeing.

Parts of Ayurveda

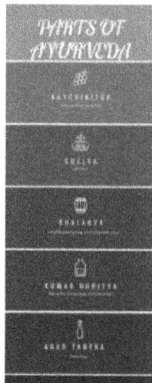

PARTS OF
AYURVEDA

KAYCHIKITSA

SHALYA

SHALAKYA

KUMAR BHRITYA

AGAD TANTRA

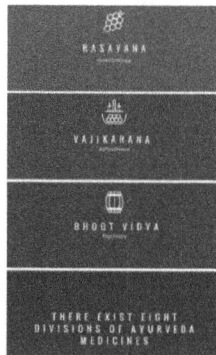

RASAYANA

VAJIKARANA

BHOOT VIDYA

THERE EXIST EIGHT
DIVISIONS OF AYURVEDA
MEDICINES

There exist eight divisions of Ayurveda medicines, to be specific

1.Kaychikitsa (Internal pharmaceutical)

2.Shalya (Surgery)

3.Shalakya (Otorhinolaryngology and Ophthalmology)

4.Kumar Bhritya (Pediatrics, Gynecology and Obstetrics)

5.Agad tantra (Toxicology)

6.Rasayana (Gerentorology)

7.Vajikarana (Aphrodisiacs)

8.Bhoot Vidya (Psychiatry)

Ayurveda Basics or Principles of Ayurveda.

Characters of life:

The coalition of body, detects, brain and soul is called life and the study of life is Ayurveda.

Pancha Mahabhuta

As indicated by the Ayurveda, It is trusted that all current living or non living matter (i.e human body) is made of Pancha Mahabhuta (five essential components)

Pancha Mahabhuta

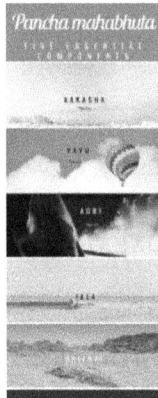

Pancha mahabhuta
FIVE ESSENTIAL COMPONENTS

AAKASHA

VAYU

AGNI

JALA

PRITHVI

1.Aakasha (The Sky)

2.Vayu The air

3.Agni  the fire

4.Jala the water

5.Prithvi the earth

Dooshas

The Dooshas are of two sorts:

1.Physical or Body Dooshas

2.Mental.

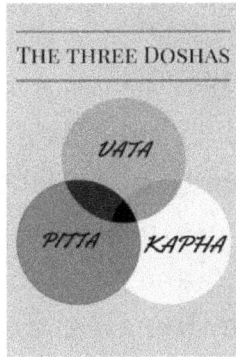

THE THREE DOSHAS

VATA

PITTA    KAPHA

There are three sorts of Doshas in the body. Doshas direct and administer a large number of partitioned capacities at the top of the priority list and body frameworks. The three Dooshas are:

Vata Dooshas

Pitta Dooshas

Kapha Dooshas

Vata Dooshas speaks to movement and stream. It is the premise of breath, dissemination and neuromuscular movement. Vata unevenness prompts blockage, uneasiness and sleep deprivation. Its central site in the body is in the Large Intestine.

Pitta Dooshas coordinates all metabolic exercises, vitality trade and processing. Pitta unevenness prompts peptic ulcers, hypertension, and incendiary inside infections, skin sicknesses and unfavorably susceptible responses. It is additionally in charge of outrage, envy and desire and its central site in the body is around the Navel locale.

Kapha Dooshas speaks to structure and attachment and liquid adjust. Kapha unevenness leads towards infections of the respiratory framework, sinusitis, diabetes mellitus, corpulence, atherosclerosis and tumors. It is additionally in charge of sentiments of connection and covetousness. Its main site in the body is in the Chest.

Whenever Vata, Pitta and Kapha, are in adjust, wellbeing is ideal and when the adjust is exasperates, medical DISEASE surface.

The easy approach to comprehend Dooshas is by its qualities. You can watch the characteristics of TriDooshas effectively in your own particular body.

The characteristics of Vata Dooshas are

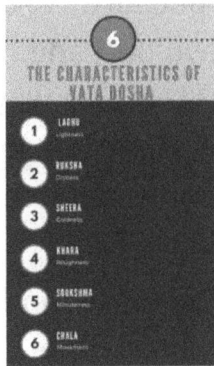

•Laghu-Lightness

•Ruksha-Dryness

•Sheera-Coldness

•Khara-Roughness

•Sookshma-Minuteness

•Chala-Movement

• Dryness – Any indication in the body that is related with dryness is impacted by Vata. For instance – Dry skin. Dry and split foot, Dry eye disorder, dry lips and so forth. All the skin ailments with dryness as a component are expected to Vata Dooshas.

•Lightness – Because Vata Dooshas is made out of Vayu (air) and Akasha (ether), it is actually light. In this way, at whatever point you feel there is softness in the body, you can aimlessly accept that Vata is affecting your body.

•Coldness – Coldness and dryness are between associated. Like, amid winter, your skin tends to feel dry. See that both cool and dry are Vata qualities. At whatever point your hands or legs are feeling chilly, you can accept that there is Vata increment. Amid winter, the impression of torment will be more. Torment is a manifestation of Vata, and coldness is expanding the Vata side effect.

•Roughness – Dryness and unpleasantness exist with each other. Like unpleasantness in lips, harsh broke foot, and so on are normal for Vata action.

•Minuteness – Vata, being made of ether and air, it can infiltrate through all the body channels, into most profound tissues.

•Chala – development – increment in development is because of Vata.

•The development of liquids, nourishment, supplements and so forth inside body, gastro intestinal track is because of Vata.

•Locomotion exercises, for example, strolling; appendage developments are because of Vata.

•Anything that is identified with development is because of Vata.

•Excretion of dung, pee and so forth are because of Vata as it were.

•Ayurveda examines three Dooshas or psyche/body administrators to keep particle adjust for ideal wellbeing. Vata is the lead Dooshas and represents all development in the body.

The characteristics of Pitta Dooshas are

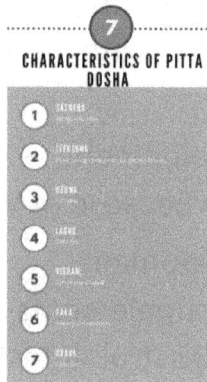

CHARACTERISTICS OF PITTA DOSHA

Sasneha – marginally slick

Teekshna – puncturing, going into profound tissues

Ushna – hotness

Laghu – delicacy

Visram –unpleasant smell

Sara – having smoothness, development

Drava – liquidity are the characteristics of Pitta.

Pitta Dooshas can be contrasted with flame.

•Slightly slick – For flame to consume, you would require some oil or ghee as fuel. In the event that you add oil to flame, the fire would increment.

•Piercing, infiltrating – Because Pitta is comprised of flame and water, it has the ability to go into profound body tissues.

•Ushna – hotness – All the warm figures the body is impacted by Pitta Dooshas. For case, processing, body temperature and so on. All the metabolic exercises additionally create some measure of vitality, and consequently are impacted by Pitta Dooshas. Whenever there is increment in temperature, as in fever, there is increment of Pitta in the body.

•Lightness – on the grounds that Pitta is made of water and fire segments, and fire part is higher than the water part, gentility is likewise a nature of Pittha.

•Bad smell — The awful breath issue is normally impacted by Pitta Dooshas. The terrible stench in excrement and pee are additionally affected by Pitta.

•Fluidity, liquidity — are additionally characteristics of Pitta. Pitta can be conceptualized as a fluid fuel consuming.

## Chapter 9: Ayurveda In Use

When to and when not to use ayurveda?

Though, there do not exist many hard-core scientific evidences to support the use of ayurvedic techniques but chances are quite fair that these can boost your energy levels, relax you and make you feel better in general thereby lowering to a great extent, your risk of some serious illness.

Whether to use ayurvedic system of medication or not is more or less a personal judgement after considering all the merits and demits of the concept. To try out with ayurveda you may have it applied on chronic but minor ailments. Remember that though it can cure diseases to an extent, ayurveda can't give you eternal vigor and life not it can rid you off cancer, diabetes or heart diseases.

Ayurveda can be described s basically a lifestyle that makes one feel better. The method of under-nutrition without malnutrition proves to be the only scientific way of prolonging life in mammals. Well...then it can also be argued that imposing any sort of discipline in life makes you feel better! Like Chinese system of medicine, ayurveda is not recommended in dealing with an acute infection such as pneumonia. Rather it should be used to supplement more conventional treatments for serious and advanced diseases like speeding up of surgical recovery or alleviating side effects of cancer treatment. One piece of advice needs mention here – never use herbs from other tradition in mixture with ayurvedic herbs without consulting some practitioner who is well versed with all of them.

Benefits And Harms Of Ayurveda

Ayurveda happens to be most useful in treatment of allergies, chronic fatigue, ulcers, rashes, indigestion, insomnia, depression and anxiety. It also helps to speed up surgical recovery and acts as supplement to conventional treatment for serious illness such as cancer.

However, some ayurvedic medicines containing heavy metals of the like of lead and mercury are poisonous no much how much heat processing they have been put through. The philosophical aspect of ayurveda at times may put you down. Though, the concept of ayurveda that people control their own destiny is all positive one, but it also projects the view that you fall sick because of your own will. That's certainly not true!

Healing The Ayurvedic Way

Some of the most common techniques of ayurvedic healing are as follows:

1)Sensory delights –

Everything you see, hear, smell, taste and feel also impacts your health to a large extent. Based on this concept are some of the ayurvedic healing techniques which ask you to surround yourself with balms for the senses including soothing music, invigorating aromas, beautiful hues, and mesmerizing massages.

2) Diet and dosha –

Each of the six tastes as recognized by ayurveda – sour, sweet, salty, pungent, bitter and astringent – has specific effect on the doshas. Based on this, the ayurvedic dietary therapy prescribes eating specific food to pacify a dosha that goes out of equilibrium. For e.g. a kapha type patient is told to avoid sweets and eat more pungent bitter and astringent foods such greens, spices, beans and potatoes.

3) Marma therapy –

According to ayurveda, internal prana masts the outer world at 107 marmas (junctions). These points which are more or less like acupuncture points, when pressed, stimulate the mind-body connection and help in equilibrating your doshas. One can get marma therapy at any ayurvedic clinic or can learn to do it by oneself.

4) Yoga asanas –

Yoga asanas are a set of postures which help to integrate mind and body. These yogic exercises can be used to stretch and activate marma points. The most commonly used is the hatha yoga which stresses physical exercises.

5) Meditation –

It is basically a method of focusing our thoughts on the silence and wisdom inside us by way of special chanting and breathing exercises. Meditation is considered as an important part of self healing since, ayurveda holds that by exploring this inner place, one can find the means to health and well being.

6) Breathing exercises –

Since ayurveda considers breathing to be a bodily expression of vital energy, many ayurvedic doctors and therapists recommend a soothing set of balanced breathing exercises called as pranayama. These breathing exercises are great source of relaxation for getting into sync with universal energies.

7) Detoxification –

Getting rid of the body toxins, which can mess up one's dosha balance thereby predisposing the body to disease, is an important aspect of ayurvedic healing. Lots of efforts is put into purging impurities via the three malas i.e. sweat, urine and faeces. For mental impurities one is needed to purge negative thoughts and feelings. Various method of purging bodily impurities includes steam bath, enema, laxative, vomiting and bloodletting. Moreover, to get the impurities out, other than inhaling medicated oils and undergoing oil massages and herbalized sweat treatments, one is supposed to endure extended periods of fasting, diarrhoea, mucous discharge, induced vomiting and occasional bloodletting.

Efficacy

Although no major scientific evidence exists to back the effectiveness of ayurvedic treatment, the practical experience of massage and relaxation has received positive response from the patients worldwide. One research on ayurvedic treatments of rheumatoid arthritis concluded that some of the reported clinical trials failed to show that ayurvedic theories are effective options for RA. Similarly a paper on use of ayurvedic treatment for cardiovascular disease concluded that there is no strong evidence to prove the effectiveness of ayurvedic medicines and therapies. But the practitioners are hopeful that further research could prove its efficiency in a more accurate manner.

Ayurveda And Cancer

Ayurveda describes different stages of tumor growth as chronic inflammatory and intractable diseases with chances of developing malignancy, probable malignancy, benign glandular swelling and definite malignancy. See the figure below.

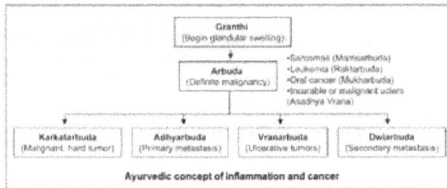

Ayurvedic concept of inflammation and cancer

Ayurvedic theory believes that cancer is a result of lifestyle errors such as unhealthy foods, poor behaviour, poor hygiene, physical trauma, lack of physical activity, all leading to disequilibrium of vata, pitta and kapha. Such disequilibrium results in the injury to the inner layer of the dermis leading to the formation of abnormal branches of blood vessels. Granthi or arbuda can develop at this stage in the form of bubble shaped glandular growths. Tridoshic tumors are usually malignant since all of the three major body humors lose mutual coordination, thus resulting in morbid condition.

The therapeutic approach within the ayurvedic concepts of treatment of cancer involves prakritistani chikitsa (health maintenance), rasayana chikitsa (spiritual approach) and roganashani chikitsa (disease cure). Treatment basically involves herbal remedies, surgical removal of tumor, dietary modifications and spiritual treatment like rejuvenation, prayers, music therapy, aromatherapy, gem therapy, yoga, meditation, etc. Ayurvedic treatment of various cancers involves a holistic approach and is widely preferred. The new developments in 'system biology' and 'genome revolution' are expected to provide a holistic approach to the treatment of cancer. But since this approach is devoid of the relationship between mind, body and spirit, ayurveda can help fill this gap.

Ayurveda And Diabetes

Diabetes is one of the eight critical diseases i.e. 'Maha Rog' in ayurveda which in total identifies 20 diseases. If the diabetes is related to Phlegm and Gall, it can be cured with right medication. On the other hand, diabetes mellitus which is related to gas usually lasts a lifetime. The only way to control it is through regular exercise, diet and excellent control of body weight. Ayurveda diagnoses diabetes by way of urine as it denotes the stage of excessive urination. A person suffering from diabetes mellitus will have reddish and sweet urine.

Diabetes can be of two types – type one - caused by genetic disorders; type two – caused due to ageing and poor lifestyle habits. Diabetes is known as 'Madhumeha' in ayurveda. It is recognized as a problem caused by aggravation of vata or air. Impairment of vata is indicated by deterioration of the body. Ayurveda basically does not consider diabetes as a disease which needs to be treated by only medicine or a dietary regimen. Rather the treatment as prescribed in ayurveda as against modern medicine, aims at rejuvenating the body to not only balance the sugar levels but also confirming that no further complication is caused due to the disease.

The ayurvedic treatment for this disease involves an entire change in the lifestyle of the patient along with proper medication and healthy diet. These changes, pertaining to lifestyle and diet helps in rejuvenating the body cells and tissues thereby aiding them to produce insulin properly. Apart from these aspects, ayurveda also considers mental aspect of diseases which helps the brain function in right manner before the medicines are administered.

Typical Visit To An Ayurvedic Physician

At the first visit, an ayurvedic doctor determines patient's prakrit or combination of doshas by way of examining pulse, tongue, nails, face, eyes, and posture as well as other lifestyle habits pertaining to eating, working, playing, sleeping, etc. He will assess the way patient's voice sounds when your answer these questions. This will be followed by a customized health plan in order to harmonize the imbalanced doshas. Such a plan prescribes specific regimen of herbs, foods, yoga, massage, asanas, exercises and meditations. This engages in the concept that you are your own healer rather than relying on someone else to do it for you.

The patient is probably put on a regular regime of rasayanas which may be a mixture of herbs, fruits, and minerals in various forms to treat specific diseases and promote good health. The patient may be asked to make some specific changes in his patterns on sleeping, eating, working, and exercising. Weeks or months later the practitioner may put the patient through certain exams in order to monitor the progress.

## Chapter 10: The Ayurvedic Way Of Life

Ayurveda for a Balanced Diet -Vata, Pitta & Kapha Doshas

Ayurveda, the ancient holistic health sister science to yoga, recognizes that health is a state of balance between the body, mind, and consciousness. In ancient times, food was considered medicine. The principles of healthy eating were well-known and the healing properties of foods and herbs were used to correct imbalances.

One of the most important aspects of the system of Ayurveda is the tridoshas, or forces that generate and maintain physical and mental health:

Vata (Air): Sustains the body and originates every kind of physical movement in the body. It controls the mind and senses and causes elimination of wastes.

Pitta (Bile): Responsible for digestion, heat, the digestive fire and the formation of blood.

Kapha (Phlegm): nourishes and lubricates the body, maintains sexual potency, and lends mental balance to the individual

The three Ayurvedic doshas, or primal metabolic tendencies, give us a great strategy for figuring out how to maintain a healthy weight. If you have too much kapha active in your body, you will add fat. Most obesity problems are the result of accumulating kapha. Pitta tends to contribute to a balanced body weight. Since this is the hot dosha, we can increase it to burn off the fat of kapha. Vata tends to favor reducing weight. When you are healthy, and your doshas are balanced, your weight will be stable.

If you are retaining water, feel sluggish and have a chest full of mucus, you may be experiencing a kapha imbalance, and should use a kapha-balancing diet until your body is again balanced and healthy. If you are hot, irritated, and have regular inflammation such as bursitis, you may be experiencing a pitta imbalance, and should use a pitta-balancing diet. If you have trouble keeping weight on, are spaced out, feel weak or exhausted, and are constipated, you may be living with a vata imbalance, and should use a vata-balancing diet.

| Overactive Dosha | Qualities | Diet Should Be | Suggested foods for balancing |
|---|---|---|---|
| Kapha | Cold, Wet, Heavy | Warm, Dry, Light | Eat low fat, low calorie, less total food; hot spices, occasional fasting, less frequency, largest meal midday. |

|  |  |  | Dry and astringent fruits (apple, raisin), Vegetables, especially raw, Dry grains (rice cakes), Hot spices (black pepper), Cooked beans with warming spices, Spicy herbal teas (ginger). Avoid Sweet fruits, Nuts, Milk products, Oil. |
|---|---|---|---|
| Pitta | Hot, Wet, | Cool, Dry, | Eat mote of sweet fruits, |

| | Light | Heavier | sweet and bitter vegetables (greens), Beans in general, Natural sweeteners (maple syrup), Mild cheeses (cottage cheese), Sweet and cooling drinks (apple juice) |
| --- | --- | --- | --- |
| | | | Avoid Sour fruits, Pungent vegetables (onion), Nuts, Hot spices, |

| | | | Fermented milk products (yogurt), Oils. |
|---|---|---|---|
| Vata | Cold, Dry, Light | Warm, Moist, Heavier | Have more of nourishing, easy to digest, warm, filling, heavy, moistening, strengthening, small frequent regular meals, mild warming spices, calm and concentrate while eating. Avoid Dry |

| | | | fruits, Dry grains (rice cakes), Raw vegetables, Cabbage family (broccoli), Beans in general, Any food which causes gas |
|---|---|---|---|
| | | | |

Personalize your Exercise Routine with Ayurveda

| For Balancing Kapha | For Balancing Pitta | For Balancing Vata |
|---|---|---|
| Get hot | Don't overheat, cool air | Stay warm |
| Sweat | Don't be fanatical - take a break | Mild only - don't overdo |

| Vigorous aerobic | Drink plenty of water | Regular routine - stick with a program |
|---|---|---|
| Work up to pushing your limits | Vary the routine to avoid boredom | Slow, gradual progress |
| Discipline | Varied overall fitness program | Walking |
| Powerful calisthenics | Moderate length workout to avoid overheating | Stretching, yoga |

Yogic Diet

Yogic diet does not include meat, fish, poultry, or eggs. You can get all the proteins, vitamins, and minerals you need without them. A yogic diet is a balanced combination of:

Fruits

Nuts

Vegetables

Grains

Legumes

Dairy products (except eggs)

Whole, fresh, unprocessed nutritious foods give you energy and strength. When your diet consists of nutritious and sustaining foods and you eat only what you know you can digest, then you are on your way to a healthy, happy, and holy life.

Have you ever wondered why people gain weight at different rates, walk at different speeds and are prone to different health problems? According to the ancient Indian healing system Ayurveda, the answer lies in your constitution type or Dosha.

What IS Dosha?

Dosha literally translates as "that which changes" and is a type of life force which determines your biological and psychological attributes. There are three basic types of Dosha: Vata, Pitta and Kapha. Although some people have one prevailing Dosha, most people are characterised by two Doshas. It's rare to be entirely Vata, Pitta or Kapha and even rarer to be all three.

VATA

Vata is considered the "leader of the Doshas" and can mimic Pitta and Kapha. It governs the movement of the body. Those who are primarily Vata type tend to be tall, thin and have trouble gaining weight. With a long slim body, prominent bone structure and a quick, light gait, Vata types often have irregular eating and sleeping patterns and feel the cold more than other Dosha types.

Vata types are talkative and learn quickly but often have trouble remembering what they have learnt and have difficulty making decisions. They are emotional by nature and their moods change quickly.

Vata imbalance can lead to digestive problems, gas, bloating and dry skin, as well as a loss of control over your activity and a racing, unfocused mind, which can lead to anxiety and depression.

The best way of balancing Vata is to seek warmth and stability, by sticking to a regular sleeping and eating schedule, wearing warm clothing in warm colors appropriate for the season and favoring soothing, calm music and sweet, heavy aromas. Light exercise which focuses on balance and flexibility, such as yoga, Tai Chai and aerobics is perfect for Vata types. Low-fat dairy products, olive oil, rice, wheat, nuts, cooked vegetables, spices and sweet heavy fruits are all recommended for pacifying Vata, however beans, barely, corn, sprouts, cabbage, raw vegetables and dry, light fruits should be avoided.

## PITTA

Feisty, driven and highly determined, Pitta types make excellent decision makers, speakers and teachers. They tend to have a well-defined body with good muscle tone, a rosy complexion, symmetrical features and find it easy to gain and lose weight. Pitta types are efficient, focused and orderly in their activities and they love a challenge! These intelligent perfectionists are very direct, sharp-witted and outspoken, however they often considered stubborn, struggle to tolerate disagreements and can be overly critical of themselves and others.

Out-of-balance pitta types are highly argumentative, short-tempered and can suffer from excessive body heat, heart burn, burning sensations and skin rashes.

To bring Pitta back into balance it is important to make choices which are calming and stabilizing. By balancing rest and activity, spending time outside surrounded by nature and making sure that they laugh many times every day, Pitta types can calm down and rediscover balance. Cool colors and light, calming aromas are also helpful. The recommended diet for Pitta types is high in dairy products, wheat, barley and rice as well as sweet fruits and cooling seasonings such as coriander, cilantro, cardamom, saffron, and fennel. Foods and flavors to avoid include hot spices and sour, acidic fruits.

## KAPHA

Kapha is the Dosha which governs the structure of the body and people with this type of Dosha tend to be soft and solid in build, with smooth skin, big eyes and full features. They have a tendency to hold on to excess weight and usually eat less frequently than Pitta types but enjoy bigger, heavier meals. With a slow metabolism and steady, measured gait, Kapha types sleep soundly and peacefully. Often described as loyal, strong, patient and caring, Kapha types make faithful friends and are able to enjoy life, as long as they stay in their comfort zone. They are often resistant to change and protective of their routine.

The physical effects of Kapha imbalance can be excessive sleep, becoming overweight, fluid retention, asthma and diabetes. Additionally, they may cling to unproductive or even destructive relationships, jobs or other comforts, which can lead to depression.

Stimulation is the best way to balance Kapha. Getting regular exercise, frequently decluttering and throwing out things that are no longer useful and favoring bright colours and stimulating aromas can help bring Kapha back into balance. Beans, ginger tea, honey, light fruits and most vegetables are great for controlling Kapha. Heavy fruits, dairy, nuts, oats, rice, wheat and sweeteners other than honey should be cut out or reduced.

## Chapter 11: Firm Breasts

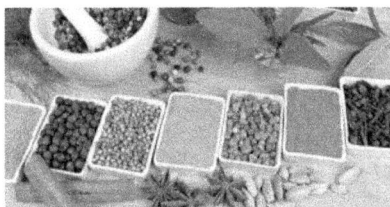

• Women tend to lose the firmness in their breasts as they age

• This generally occurs at a younger age for women who have large breasts

Symptoms to look for:

• Sagging breasts

Causes:

• Ageing

• Breastfeeding

• Loss of weight

Natural home remedy using egg and onion:

1. Take the white of an egg

2. Beat it into a cream

3. Apply this cream on the bottom of your breasts

4. Leave it for 30 min

5. Chop and crush 1 onion

6. Press the crushed onion on a sieve to extract juice

7. Add the juice to 1 glass water

8. Wash off the cream with this water

Natural home remedy using fenugreek powder:

1. Fenugreek has properties, which help the breast grow and be firm.

2. Take ¼ bowl of fenugreek powder

3. Add water

4. Mix well to make paste

5. Massage this paste on your breast

6. Leave it for 5 min

7. Wash off with water

Tips:

• Swimming is a great exercise to have firm breasts. It strengthens the pectoral muscles

Menstrual Problems:

• Production of hormones like estrogen and progesterone trigger the development of a woman's body

• Menstruation is a natural process and women experience various problems before and during

menstruation

Symptoms to look for:

• Abdominal cramps

• Pain

• Excessive flow

• Sudden stoppage

• Development of clots

Natural home remedy using papaya:

1. Papaya helps to reduce the pain and regulates the flow

2. Take pulp of an unripe papaya

3. Blend it with 1 glass water

4. Drink it twice a day

Natural home remedy using sesame seeds:

1. Sesame seeds have pain relieving properties and also cure vomiting

2. Crush 4 tsp of sesame seeds into powder

3. Add 1 glass of water

4. Mix well

5. Drink 2 times a day

Tips:

• Avoid caffeine

• Drink 8 glasses of water everyday to keep the body hydrated

Leucorrhea (Leucorrhoea):

• Leucorrhea refers to a condition wherein there's a whitish discharge from a woman's vagina

• It is commonly known as whites

• This usually happens during intervals between menstruation cycles

• Usually lasts from a week to months

- If not treated, it can turn chronic in nature

Symptoms to look for:

- Whitish discharge from vagina

- Discharge is thick with pungent odour

- Weakness

- Lower back pain

- Painful calves

- Abdominal discomfort

- Constipation

- Headaches

- Excessive itching

Causes:

- Damage to cervix during childbirth

- When the body is unable to remove toxins from the body with help of skin, bowels, lungs or the kidneys, the

toxins are removed via the mucous membrane of the uterus and vagina

Natural home remedy using coriander seeds:

1. Soak 3 tbsp coriander seeds in 1 cup water overnight

2. Strain this mixture in the morning

3. Drink this on an empty stomach

Natural home remedy using lady fingers and honey:

1. Cut 100 gm fresh lady fingers along their length

2. Boil them in 1 L water for 20 min

3. Strain and collect the water

4. Add 1 tbsp honey to the water

5. Mix well

6. When lukewarm, drink 60-90 ml doses regularly

Tips:

• Drink 1 glass of cranberry juice 2-3 times daily

• Eat 2-3 bananas and follow it with 1 tsp of clarified butter daily

Menstrual Cramps:

• Menstrual cramps refer to the throbbing pain which occurs at the onset or during a menstrual period

Causes:

• Prostaglandin is a hormone like substance, which leads to contraction of the uterus muscles and cause abdominal pain

Natural home remedy using flaxseeds:

1. Eat 2 tbsp of flaxseeds every day during periods

2. This reduces prostaglandin levels in the body

Natural home remedy using ginger, honey, lemon and tea:

1. Prepare black tea

2. Add to it ½ tsp of crushed ginger

3. Add 2 tsp lemon juice

4. Add 1 tsp honey

5. Drink this tea at regular intervals during the day

Natural home remedy using basil leaves:

1. Crush a handful of basil leaves

2. Press the paste on a sieve to extract juice

3. Take 1 glass hot water

4. Add 2 tsp basil leave juice

5. Mix well

6. Drink thrice everyday

Tips:

• Acupuncture treatment provides pain relief

• Include in diet:

  o Cinnamon

  o Sesame seeds

  o Ginger

  o Parsley

# Chapter 12: Ayurvedic Body Types

As per the science of Ayurveda, each individual has a basic 'prakriti' or characteristic. Any disease and its cure, and health of a human body as per ayurveda is governed by the 3 Doshas (a terminology is ayurveda) they are namely:

§

§Vata

§Pita

§Kapha

'Dosha' literally means that which are not correct or have the ability to go out of balance. Ayurveda states that our body consists of basically the following five elements:

Earth (Prthvi),

Water (Jala),

Fire (Agni),

Air (Vayu), and

Sky (Akasa)

The three 'doshas' mentioned above could be combined into about 10 possible combinations which is like arriving at 10 possible behavior and body types. It is interesting to note here that:

"Vata" ayurvedic body type have in them the air and space elements

"Pitta"ayurvedic body type consist of fire and water elements

§ "Kapha" ayurvedic body type comprise of earth and the water elements

Why should you care to know which ayurvedic body type you are?

Believe it or not, according to ayurvedic texts, each body on this planet earth is comprised of some unique combinations of the 'doshas' mentioned above.

If one intends to follow an ayurvedic treatment for some disease, one needs to know affirm what kind of body type he/she has as per ayurveda. The correct treatment would not be rendered otherwise. A balance is in the tree elements "vata, pitta and kapha" is necessary for a human body to function effectively without any ailments.

These are also known to be Tridoshas (a Sanskrit terminology). These have the ability to direct the metabolic and physiological activities in a human body.You would not have to see a doctor if you come across a good ayurvedic centre for your regular ailments.

The medicines that ayurveda provides has benefits and have tested to be miraculous some times. Each body is different and as such, it is indispensable to determine which body type one has in ayurvedic terms.

Additional insight - It is not just the imbalance of doshas as per ayurveda which causes diseases. The tridoshas are actually the primary disease causing elements. Other than these there are few factors which cause diseases and are secondary factors in getting a disease in human beings. These are as follows:

Body tissues (or the dhatus)

The toxins (or the ama)

The waste materials (or the malas)

Having said all this, knowing your body type as per the ayurvedic terms helps you create a diet chart as per your personal body type. The ayurvedic centres prompt to get some personal special diets or lifestyle changes to get over with any diseases or just to de - stress lives.

Elaborating upon the ayurvedic body types:

Vata type body – This body type would show enhanced characteristics of physical and emotional stature. As stated earlier these body types comprise of air and space elements. The general body structure of a vata body type people would be lean and thin. They would have difficulty in gaining weight.

It is to be noted that it is an imbalance in vata which in turn disorders all irrespective of the body type one will be prone to have some ailments. A balance of this 'dosha' is quite essential in every human being as per ayurvedic texts. This body type moment is exceptionally quick, however with have poor retention capacity.

Pitta type body – Pitta type people have a normal medium kind of a body. However they would generally have thin hair and are prone to either hair loss or baldness. They sleep sound but when they talk they like to do it loud with dominance. Intelligence quotient is found to be on the higher side.

Kapha type body - Kapha type body are generally obese strong white teeth. However their digestion is comparatively slower. Kapha type people are found to be emotional. They probably because of this nature tend to forgive soon. Intelligence is found to be medium.

Note: the words mentioned in brackets are the actual technical terminologies used in Sanskrit language in which ayurveda is actually conceived.

## Chapter 13: Weight Loss

Are you serious about weight loss, but at the same-sex time want to improve overall health? Then opting for ayurveda is the best answer. Today I would like to share the quick fix Ayurveda alterations that you can make to your lifestyle to help with sustained weight-loss.

Before knowing more about weight loss through Ayurveda, let's understand Ayurveda first. Ayurveda is derived from two Sanskrit words Ayur and Veda. Ayur means life or longevity, while veda means Science. In other words, Ayurveda is a Science of Life. Originated in India, an ancient medicine system, which has now gained scientific backing for most methods, unlike other conventional methods.

Does Ayurveda Really Help With Weight Loss?

Without a doubt, it does help with weight loss, or dealing with any other health problem for that matter. Besides, Ayurveda deals with identifying and treating the root cause of the problem, resulting in a permanent solution.

Ayurveda has underlying principles for every problem, with all the diseases being classified under different body types. There's no universal solution in Ayurveda and the medicines are suggested based on one's body type, problems, symptoms and various other factors. There are several Ayurvedic medicines for weight loss, which you can try. It is important to understand it is not a quick fire solution, rather, effective and comprehensive weight loss aids that offer definitive benefits slowly but steadily. The best part is that, the weight lost using Ayurvedic methods are permanent, as long as you adhere to the suggestions.

Tips To Follow During Weight Loss With Ayurveda:

Before going into the medicines, let us take a look at the suggestions for maintaining ideal body, and tips to follow during weight loss efforts.

Early To Bed And Early To Rise:

The principal tip is to sleep early and rise early. The best time to hit the bed is 10 PM, at most 11PM, and rising at 5 AM or by 6 AM is a must. Our body functions in an organized way in line with nature and adhering to the natural cycle, works the best. Our body functions active during the day and rests at night. When we follow this routine, many health problems, including obesity is tackled naturally.

Three Meals:

Eating three meals is ideal, unless you have low blood sugar levels. Having multiple meals is not advised in Ayurveda, unlike what many health care professionals claim today. Instead, a healthy breakfast, scrumptious lunch and a light dinner are recommended. Our liver is at its best during noon, so your heavy meal should be at noon. This way, the body assimilates what is ingested. Also, for healthy and natural detoxification, our liver should have enough rest at night (to detoxify the body), a reason why dinner should be light.

Go Natural:

Nature has everything we need, though we hardly realize it. Seasonal fruits and veggies are for a reason. Our body needs food according to the different seasons and that's why, our body craves seasonal foods during those seasons. Besides staples like rice, wheat and other fruits and veggies, seasonal fruits and veggies should be part of our diet during their respective seasons.

Water:Lastly, drinking water soon after or before a meal is not advisable. While water is good for overall health and weight loss, consuming it with food dilutes stomach acids that aid with digestion. This is the reason many are obese, since food is not broken down or assimilated properly. Built-up toxins, hormonal imbalance, improper digestion, etc. are just a few contributing factors of weight gain and obesity. On the contrary, sipping water throughout the day, in particular, warm water is ideal and aids with digestion and detoxification.

Now that the most confusing concepts are cleared, let's move on Ayurvedic medicines for weight loss.

1. Lemon & Honey:

The most common remedy is lemon with honey. Every morning, the first thing you consume right after brushing should be warm water with lemon juice and honey. This is a delicious drink too! This potent combo reduces appetite, detoxifies the body and aids with weight loss without affecting your health. Many fear lemons, due to cold. If you fear so, you can use hot water to combat it.

2. Pepper:

While lemon and honey will do the trick, adding pepper powder makes it more potent. Though it is not a compulsion to have early morning, you can have it once during the day. Also, if you fear lemons are going to give a cold, the pepper will combat it!

3. Cabbage:

Cabbage can be consumed raw, or cooked. When it's raw, it is more potent. Eat a bowl of cabbage every day to boost fat burning. You can have it before food, or substitute it as a snack.

4. Digestive Aids:

Weight gain is often due to improper digestion, or lack of digestion fire according to Ayurveda. Increasing foods that increase digestive fire works wonders with weight loss. Foods that boost digestion and enhance your digestive fire include ginger, papaya, bitter gourd, garlic, chilli, etc.

5. Spice Up Your Food:

Lack of spice can reduce digestion fire. Pungent, bitter and astringent foods are important for retaining digestion fire in one's body. Adding cumin, cayenne, mustard and pepper are ideal. You can substitute pepper for chilli in most recipes, or combine both. It is important to understand pepper does not aggravate acidity, rather it cools down, unlike chilli.

## 6. Get Rid Of Ama:

Ama is the term used to denote the byproduct of incomplete digestion in Ayurveda. Accumulated ama clogs lymph channels and triggers weight gain, besides leaving an individual tired. Without getting rid of it, it is difficult to deal with weight gain. Hence, consuming foods that aid with elimination of ama is important. Turmeric, Triphala (a potent combination of amalaki, haritaki and bibbitaki), trikatu (a potent combination of ginger, Indian long pepper and ginger in equal proportion), Barberry and Guggulu, all help in eliminating ama. You get these in capsule form, and you can also use powders.

## 7. Fasting:

Fasting once a week is recommended in Ayurveda for detoxification and efficient functioning of digestive system. You can have water, green teas (ginger tea, tulsi tea, mint tea, etc) and clear vegetable soups..

8. Concoction:

Mix Kutki (Scrophulariaceae), chitrak (Plumbago zeylonica) and trikatu in equal proportions. Blend well and have about ½ spoon of this mixture with a gulp of warm water. You need to swish this mixture once and then swallow. Have it once a day if you are overweight, and twice if you are obese or morbidly obese.

9. Herbs:

Other common herbs suggested in Ayurveda for weight loss include Haritaki, Bibhitaki, Amalaki, Licorice, Tulsi, Aloe Vera, Vrikshamla, etc. Most of these herbs are now available in capsule form for ease of use.

10. Ginger:

Consuming fresh ginger, with or without honey is also suggested to burn fat in Ayurveda. You could have this in the morning, since it increases body heat.

## 11. Horse Gram:

Many Ayurvedic experts suggest horse gram when you want to lose weight. You have to soak a cup of horse gram overnight, and boil it around afternoon. Once cooked, add chopped onions and rock salt to taste. Take this for 45 days, without skipping even one day! Follow this with a glass of buttermilk and see how fat is burned steadily.

## 12. Aloe Punch:

Another way is to prepare a drink with Aloe juice, turmeric powder, cumin powder, Tinospora cordifolia Powder and Terminalia Chebula Powder, in a glass of water. You can use warm water, as well. Add a spoon of honey to taste and drink it. Wait for at least one hour, before you eat anything. You can continue this drink till you lose adequate weight.

Here Are The Measurements To Prepare Aloe Punch:

Turmeric Powder: a pinch

Cumin Seeds Powder – a pinch

Aloe Vera Juice – 1 – 2 Tbsp

Tinospora cordifolia Powder – a pinch

Terminalia Chebula Powder – a pinch

13. Digestive Tea:

Take equal quantity of cumin seeds, coriander seeds and fennel seeds. About ½ spoon should do for one person. Now, add this to a bowl of water and bring it to a boil. Close the lid and boil for about five minutes. Transfer it into a flask and keep sipping it during the day. This tea will aid with digestion and weight loss.

14. Six Tastes:

Foods are classified based on their taste, namely astringent, sour, bitter, salty, sweet and pungent (spicy). It is important to ensure you get all these tastes every day, for proper functioning of the digestive system and for weight management. So remember to include a variety of foodstuffs to ensure you get all tastes and nutrients.

Ayurveda advocates almost a vegan diet for staying fit and healthy. While they don't advocate skipping meat altogether, consumption is considerably less. Besides, all processed foods and overcooked or fried foods are to be avoided.

So start skipping refined salt and sugar and find natural and healthy substitutes like rock salt, honey, licorice extract, etc. When you follow these tips religiously, besides adopting the above given remedies that are available, weight management will become a reality.

## Chapter 14: Ayurveda regime For Winter depression

Ayurveda regime for winter depression Long nights, short days, sweaters, warm clothes and chilly weather make many of us sick and depressed. This depression which surfaces especially in winter is a Seasonal Affective Disorder (SAD) and is often called as winter Time Blues or Winter depression. The exact cause for this depression is as of yet unclear. But yet few scientists believe lack of exposure to sunlight as the reason for this disorder. The symptoms of winter depression are tendency to over eat, craving for carbohydrates and sweets and weight gain. Had our ancestors observed this change in humans?

The answer is yes. Have they recommended any remedies? Yes, they have recommended simple and effective natural remedies to overcome Seasonal Affective Disorder. They have laid down explicit guidelines about diet and lifestyles which have to be followed according to seasons. The winter season is marked as Hemanta ritu and Sisira ritu in ayurveda. Hemanta ritu starts from mid November and ends in mid January. This falls in southern solstice which is called as visarga kala or dakshinayana in ayurveda. Sisira ritu starts from mid January and lasts till middle of march. Sisira ritu falls in Northern solstice which is called as Aadana kaala or uttaraayana. The response of human body to this season is very well explained in ayurveda. People will have increased strength and their digestion capacity is increased .This is marked by increased hunger. These symptoms are caused by increased body fire which is supported by vata.

Vata inside body increases in winter because of cold and dryness which is prevalent in outer atmosphere. The winter time depression is noticed mostly in persons who have vata as major constituent in their prakriti or body constitution. The cause for this type of change is longer nights of winter. Light therapy is recommended by doctors for winter time blues. Exposure to artificial light may cause headache , Irritability ,Eye strain , Inability to sleep and fatigue. Exposure to sunlight and if sunlight is not available sitting near fireplace is the remedy suggested in Ayurveda. Keeping the home well lit with lights help to reduce the intensity of depression. Moderate exercise like yoga is another remedy for winter depression. Ayurveda recommends oil massage (abhyanga) to body and head (moordha taila.). Indulging in sexual act to keep the moods elevated and to keep the body warm is another strongly suggested ayurvedic remedy. Meeting friends who are kind and understanding boosts morale and brightens up the day. Spending time with friends on the beach helps to expose your body to sunlight and keeps your spirits high. Relaxing with meditation, massage , light music and laughter helps to great extent. The following ayurvedic tips help to prevent and reduce the intensity of seasonal disorder of winter, the winter time blues.

1. Expose yourself to sunlight as much as you can. In absence of sun light sitting near fire place is very helpful.

2. Massage your body with vata balancing herbal oil (abhyanga). Never forget to apply oil on your head (moordha taila.).

3. Then remove the oil by taking hot water bath. A mixture of flours of yellow gram (channa), green gram (moong) , fenu greek seeds (methi) in equal proportion is the best herbal scrub which can be used to remove the oil. This mixture prevents the washing of natural oil from skin.

4. Consume hot soups.

5. Use vata balancing foods like wheat, oil, corn, black gram and jaggery.

6. Tickle your taste buds with sweet, sour and salt tastes

7. Always use hot water for all daily routine activity.

8. Use thick blankets and sheets made of cotton, silk and wool.

9. Always wear foot wear.

10. Indulge in sexual act.

11. Spend your leisure time with friends and relatives whom you like.

## Chapter 15: Ayurveda And Insomnia

An ayurvedic diet will help you to be mindful of what you eat, and avoid processed foods to balance the doshas and thereby help to maintain a healthy body. Remember that you should eat seasonal fruits and vegetables so that you're in tune with nature. As mentioned earlier each body type has to avoid certain foods. For example a pitta dosha body type should only take citrus fruits during day time and avoid them after sunset.

Always eat seasonal fruits and vegetables as they are in tune with nature. Try to add astringent and bitter taste to balance nutrition.

Sweet taste is good for kapha but an over dose of sweet can cause imbalance. So you need to know your body type and eat accordingly.

Foods to avoid for Pitta body types

Pitta body type should also avoid fried foods and fermented foods.

- Chips
- soda
- cola
- coffee
- spicy foods and
- oily stuff are a definite no, no.

Foods to eat for pitta body types

They should eat more of organic and natural foods that are fresh and easily digestible.

- Salads
- Soups
- Steamed vegetables
- Fruits like avocado and pears and
- Coconut oil is ideal for pitta body types.
- Eat more vegetables and less of starch.

To balance the three doshas in the body include sweet stuff, acidic and bitter taste in your diet. Drink warm milk with ginger and cardamom into it.

Foods to avoid for vata body types

• Crunchy foods

• Cold drinks

• Spicy foods

• Chickpeas

• Beans

• Leafy vegetables

• Artichokes

• Cayenne pepper

• Chilli pepper

• White sugar

As far as possible avoid fried stuff and nuts. They can cause imbalance in vata body types.

Foods to eat for vata body types

• Soft food

• Warm drinks like ginger tea

• Wheat

• Rice

- Cereals
- Almost all vegetables and fruits
- Natural sweetener like honey
- Beef, chicken, eggs and fish

Foods to avoid for kapha body types

- Fried foods
- Cold drinks/ Icecream
- Tofu
- Cheese
- Brown rice

Foods to eat for kapha body types

- Low fat milk
- Honey
- Beans
- Grains
- Vegetables

## Chapter 16: The Three Doşas

[Note I use here the "ş" with the cedilla in lieu of one with a dot beneath it, because there was not one available in my word processor. I do not know whether or not the pronunciation would be the same.]

Ayurveda conceives of 3 energies working in each person. In English, these energies are called "humours, and in Sanskrit they are called "doşas.

The concept of "humours" was part of Western medicine until recently.

Western medicine conceives of 4 humours.

In both the "doşas" model and the "humours" model, distempers (diseases) happen when, and only when, one of the types of energy is either excessive, insufficient, or "aggravated.

"Aggravated" can be understood to mean that the energy is distorted in some fashion. It is not functioning harmoniously, as it ought to do.

When all the types of energy are unblocked, unimpaired, and not excessive, then the subject is in a state of health, or wholeness. Thus it is, that a main goal or consideration of ayurvedic medicine is to put the 3 doşas into balance and harmony.

Each doşa has a distinctive character, that is to say, each one produces its own type of person, of personality in a person. Each person is naturally predominant in one or two of the doşas from the time of their birth.

Following is a list of the 3 doşas, the quality of each one, the type of person each doşa produces, and the type of illness when that doşa is excessive or aggravated:

Kapha doşa– Kapha is the sluggish energy. It is like matter, like earth or stone. It is static, inert, dull, sensual, and of small awareness.

Kapha folks are very connected to matter and the material plane, and so they naturally tend to acquire money and to be able to accumulate it.

When you see someone who has strong kapha energy, you will find that they are slow, steady, and enduring. They pick things up slowly, I mean mental things, and once they understand and learn them, they retain them.

They are possessive, and attached to keeping things the way they are, the way they are used to them.

They like to feel that they own things. Sometimes kapha folks can envy others their possessions.

Emotionally they are loving and forgiving. They will allow you to believe whatever you believe and still accept you even if they don't agree with you, given that you don't threaten their stability and security.

They are calm people, indeed. Since they are so calm, they are able to endure more stress with less effect on their bodies and their attitude, than the rest of people are able to do. Under stress, they can last a long time without and stick with it and hold out.

Pitta doşa— Pitta is the active energy of desire and ambition. It is turbulent, intense, and focused.

Pitta folks are stirred by fiery emotions.

You can see the symptoms when they need more balance in their lifestyles, when their pitta energy becomes too intense: if they get jealous, if they resent, if they get mad, if they needle, if they speak hurtfully, then they need to balance their lifestyles more than what they are doing.

It is great to have them as your friend. They are very conscientious toward their foes.

Pitta folks react to stress and challenges by "sticking to their guns".

They like to devise ways and means of getting things done, despite contrary circumstances. They are action people, with a lot of energy to get things done. Because of their focus on action, they become capable at doing things.

Pitta makes people to have courage. They will respond in kind to competition.

Pitta folks like to be straightforward in telling you clearly what they mean.

Vata doşa– Vata is the mental energy of the nerves. It is awake and alert, and mentally active.

Vata people are in constant motion. They are restless. They can become overexcited. Afterward they become extremely tired. Unless they take breaks often they become nervous and anxious. Special attention is needed for them to prevent themselves from anxiety, from worrying, or from fearing.

RECIPES

Here are a few drinks that can help you to sleep well at night. These drinks suit all doshas.

Bed time drink

Ingredients:

• ¼ tspn Nutmeg Powder

• 2 tspn Honey

Instructions:

Add 1-2 drops of water to the Nutmeg powder followed by honey and mix it thoroughly into a paste and set aside.

Bring 1 cup of water to a boil.

Turn off the heat and add the nutmeg paste to the water and stir well.

Consume while hot.

This will induce good sleep as the warm water relaxes the insides of your body and makes you feel drowsy. You can also substitute water with milk.

Poppy seed serum

Ingredients:

- 1 tspn poppy seeds.
- 1 cup milk
- 1 tbspn Honey
- A pinch of cardamom powder
- A pinch of nutmeg powder

Instructions:

Make the poppy seeds into a powder using grinder.

Bring 1 cup of milk to a boil.

Add the poppy seed powder and let it simmer for 1-2 minutes.

Turn off the heat.

Add cardamom powder, nutmeg powder and Honey to the milk

Mix thoroughly and drink while hot.

Consume it before going to bed.

Breakfast drink

Ingredients:

- 1 ½ cup of Milk
- 7-8 Almonds, soaked in water for 8/9 hours and finely chopped. (instead of

soaked almonds you can also use blanched almonds in case you forget to soak them.)

- 5-6 Dates, deseeded and finely chopped
- ½ tspn of Cinnamon powder
- ½ tspn of Cardamom powder
- ¼ tspn of Turmeric powder
- ¼ tspn of Nutmeg powder
- 1 ½ tbspn of Ghee (Clarified Butter)
- 2-3 Black Peppercorns (crushed)

Instructions:

Add all the ingredients to the milk and stir thoroughly till the spice powders are mixed well.

Put this mixture in a blender to get thick consistency for the mixture.

Try to soak the almonds the previous night in water. In case you've forgotten don't fret. Just keep it in microwave for 2 minutes and remove the outer skin. It'll peel off easily.

Ayurvedic Breakfast Serum

Ingredients:

146

- 1 ½ cup of Milk

- 4-5 Almonds, soaked overnight and finely chopped

- 5-6 Dates, deseeded and finely chopped

- ½ cup of grated Coconut or Coconut flakes

- ½ tspn of Cardamom powder

- ¼ tspn of Nutmeg powder

- 2 tbspn of Ghee (Clarified Butter)

- 2 tbsps of Honey

Instructions:

Add all the ingredients (except Honey) to the milk and stir thoroughly till the spice powders are mixed well.

Put this mixture in a blender to get thick consistency for the mixture.

After blending bring this mixture to a boil and then let it simmer for 2-3 minutes.

Turn off the heat.

Watermelon and mint juice for pitta

Ingredients

- Watermelon fruit
- Mint leaves
- Piece of ginger
- ½ lemon
- Sweetener

Instructions

Cut cubes of watermelon pieces into the blender along with a few mint leaves. Add a slice of ginger and one half of lemon juice. Blend everything together along with a sweetener. Strain the liquid and keep it to cool. This juice will help to remove the toxins and balance the pitta.

## Chapter 17: A Healthy Life Through The Ayurveda Diet

Will you agree with the statement "you are what you eat?" If that's the case, then if you eat a lot of delicious but unhealthy foods, then what does it mean? That you are an unhealthy person? I don't think you would want yourself to reflect an unhealthy lifestyle, and most especially, you would not want to become unhealthy right? By the end of this paper, you will be informed of a healthy diet through Ayurveda ways. A good diet is still one of the best ways to live a healthy life.

Before anything else, what first is Ayurveda? Ayurveda, meaning "science of life," is a form of alternative medicine which believes that imbalance and disturbances in the body's natural energy causes diseases and other health problems. Ayurvedic principles state that a person is made up of three doshas or basic life energy forces. These doshas live in harmony and balance with each other but when something disturbs that balance, problems kick in. Treatment in Ayurveda is unlike our usual ways. In conventional medicine, we treat the symptoms of the problem. In other alternative medicines, the physiological cause of the problem is addressed. In Ayuverdic medicine, treatments are geared towards reestablishing balance of the doshas. How? One is through Ayurveda diet.

Ayurveda diet can be done by everyone. It does not require a specific age, nor is it limited to people who have health problems. Depending on what type of dosha you have and what dosha is causing the imbalance, your diet can be altered to restore the balance. Wait. Maybe you are thinking "I thought 3 doshas live in harmony?" Yes. You are right. But one of the doshas is more dominant with the others as this determines the type of your personality. Ayuverdic practitioners' first step is determining if you are a Vatta,

Kapha, or Pitta then where you are having imbalance with. From there, they could formulate a treatment plan for you. The following are tips you could use if you want to introduce and slowly make Ayuverdic diet part of your lifestyle:

• Start with replacing your refrigerator's contents. Replace processed foods with fresh and healthy ones.

• Go for foods that are suited for your doshas.

• To promote balance of your Vata, sweet, salty, sour, heavy, oily, and hot foods are recommended. Examples of good food for you are chicken, almonds, bananas, lemons, cucumber, potatoes, and rice.

• For the balancing of Pitta, cold, heavy, dry, sweet, and bitter ones are good. Examples of recommended food are watermelons, mangoes, broccoli, barley, white rice, cottage cheese, and freshwater fish.

• When trying to balance the Kapha, go for foods that are punget, light, dry, hot, and bitter. Examples of food for the Kapha diet are garlic, egg plant, ghee, and ginger.

• Add herbs and spices. Doing so will aid in your digestion and in cleansing of your body.

• Always include at least a minimum amount of each of the basic tastes. These are astringent, pungent, salty, bitter, sour, and sweet.

• When eating, sit down on a comfortable place. It is best if you eat in an environment that makes you feel calm.

You see, these basic concepts of Ayurveda diet is easy to do. What more if a practitioner will guide you in doing these steps? Remember, a healthy diet will not only balance your dosha and prevent or cure certain health problems It will also let you live a happier and a longer life.

What Is Ayurveda Diet?

Ayurveda has been in great demand for the total well being of a person. Ayurveda uses all natural herbal products for the meditation process and include various other activities including yoga to bring in a balance to the whole body system of a man. Ayurveda has also considered the importance of a healthy diet to restore the essential nutrients and balance of the body. Our body can be classified into Doshas and depending on these the food constituents can be grouped accordingly. Some food that is beneficial to a particular Dosha can be harmful to another and this depends on each person's health conditions. In ayurveda ideal food is considered the main constituent for a balanced body and this requires food with lots of proteins, vitamins, minerals, fiber content and carbohydrates as the source of energy.

The Tridoshas are the Vata Dosha, Pitta Dosha and Kapha Dosha. Each Dosha has some particular qualities. Here we are discussing each Dosha and how to counterpart them with a ayurveda diet. Vata Dosha includes traits like cold, dehydrated, stiff and jagged. There are certain components that can neutralize the effects of Vata Dosha. A person suffering from Vata Dosha is recommended to have lots of diary and as well as sweet and oily foods to balance the tissue and muscles of the body. There are lots of food substances that can balance the Vata Dosha and to name some include the ghee, rice, corn and all sweet fruits. Besides that there are certain foods that can exaggerate the Dosha and these include refined oils and bad habits including smoking, consuming alcohol, junk food, spices, etc.

Pitta Dosha has the qualities like hot and oily. To balance the Dosha you need to have cool food that can smooth the body temperature and benefit the whole body system. The person has to consume lots of milk, mild spices like coriander and olive oil that are good to pita people. The foods that this person should avoid include fried and spicy foods.

Kapha Dosha has properties like cold and oily. These people have to include more light and dry food. Foods that have a bitter taste including puffed rice and leafy greens are recommended. Kapha imbalance can develop diseases like lung disorders and other heart diseases so these people have to consume lots of dry fruits.

Following healthy food habits is mandatory to be active and healthy all the time. Ayurveda diet insists on having food at moderate quantities and certain intervals of time. The food has to be consumed at a moderate rate and drink a lot of water. The ayurveda diet includes lots of fruits and vegetables that provide fiber and carbohydrates that can provide all the nutrients to the body and increase the stamina of the body. Drinking water between meals is a bad habit and ayurveda strictly prohibits this habit.

Regular exercise including yoga can rejuvenate your mind and body and relax your body functioning. Ayurvedic diet has to be practiced by every human being to lead a healthy life.

www.ingramcontent.com/pod-product-compliance
Lightning Source LLC
Chambersburg PA
CBHW060232030426
42335CB00014B/1424